Pegan Diet

Scrumptious And Welcoming Recipes For Improving
Your Health, Enhancing Well-Being, Achieving Rapid
Weight Loss, And Nurturing Your Body

*(Featuring Quick And Effortless Meals That Are
Guaranteed To Delight The Palate)*

I0090009

Calvin St-Laurent

TABLE OF CONTENT

What Is The Pegan Diet?

Are you familiar with the pegan diet? It appears rather unconventional, eliciting thoughts of the vegetarian diet... or perhaps the paleolithic diet? Undoubtedly, in accordance with its nomenclature, the pegan diet represents a harmonious amalgamation of elements derived from both the paleo diet and the vegetarian diet, striving to amalgamate the principles of these two dietary approaches and thereby surpassing the merits of both. It may seem highly unusual, given that adherents of the paleo diet are expected to consume only elemental foods that were obtainable during the ancient paleolithic era, such as vegetables, fruits, nuts, fish, and meat. This dietary approach excludes dairy, grains, sugar, oils, along with other comparable items including legumes, or even alcohol and coffee, as these were not present in that historical epoch. Conversely, the vegetarian diet dictates the strict avoidance of animal products or by-products, encompassing meats, fish, eggs, cheese, and other analogous substances, specifying the consumption solely of plant-based foods.

Consequently, individuals may find themselves significantly bewildered by the pegan diet due to its fragmented characteristics. Nevertheless, the pegan diet aims to incorporate particular principles from both diets, guidelines which will be discussed extensively at a later point. Nevertheless, the fundamental concept of the pegan diet revolves around consuming nutrient-rich whole foods, which can effectively reduce inflammation, stabilize blood sugar levels, and promote optimal health. It is evident that the pegan diet incorporates elements of both vegetarian and paleo diets, which are both restrictive in nature. It could be inferred that this suggests some flexibility in combining the two, leading to a highly restricted dietary regimen. Nevertheless, notwithstanding this notion, it is even less restrictive compared to either the vegetarian or the paleo diet alone, as it aims to incorporate principles rather than mere limitations.

Consider the alternative phrasing: "Considerable emphasis is placed on the consumption of fruits and vegetables, as evident in the vegan diet. However, in contrast to the vegan diet, the incorporation of animal proteins such as meats and fish is permissible, in addition to select nuts, seeds, and legumes." While some items that are forbidden by both diets are indeed allowed, such as certain oils and processed sugars, it is important to emphasize that the consumption of these should be greatly restricted. The pegan diet is not a haphazard or unintentional dietary approach, but rather a structured eating regimen designed to be easily adhered to.

offers the ability to persist indefinitely on it, instead of succumbing to a loss of determination to continue at a later time.

What are the fundamental principles of the Pegan Diet?

Now that we have acquired a fundamental understanding of the constituents of a legitimate pegan diet, let us now shift our focus towards examining the principles or guidelines that underpin the pegan diet. These are principles that must be familiarized with, as it can be rather perplexing to solely rely on the instruction. Taking all factors into consideration, it is evident that a vegetarian diet is unequivocal; one is able to consume foods derived from plants. The paleo diet is fundamentally straightforward: individuals should consume unprocessed, organic foods. In any event, due to the distinctive and specific nature of a pegan diet, coupled with its lesser degree of restrictiveness, the boundaries and guidelines may not be readily apparent.

Direct your attention towards adopting a predominantly plant-based dietary approach.

The fundamental concept is that it is advisable to generally adopt a diet predominantly consisting of plant-based foods. However, as previously stated, while the use of animal proteins is permissible, the majority of one's dietary intake should consist of plant-based sources. To be perfectly honest, an appropriate principle to adhere to is to ensure that at least half, if not a majority, of one's plate is occupied by vegetables at the foundation. The World Health Organization recommends a daily intake of approximately seven to eight cups of fruits and vegetables, which would serve as a commendable initial guideline. In any event, excessive consumption of certain plant-based food options should be avoided. Certain types of foods, such as starchy vegetables like potatoes and squash, should be consumed in moderation, while the predominant portion of the vegetable intake should consist of leafy greens. Taking all factors into account, one of the objectives of this dietary plan is to regulate an individual's blood sugar levels. This necessitates prioritizing consumption of low glycemic index foods, while completely rejecting foods high in simple carbohydrates and those with a high glycemic index, as they would defeat the purpose. Furthermore, there is a need to restrict natural products as well, using the same criteria applied to the limitation of generic vegetables. Notwithstanding this point, this suggestion primarily caters to individuals who still grapple with being overweight and have a more pressing need to regulate their blood sugar levels. In the absence of any glucose-related concerns, the consumption of most natural products is permissible. If an individual is experiencing difficulties in managing their glucose levels, it is advisable for them to consume mainly low-glycemic index fruits. More sugary fruits should be considered an occasional indulgence, akin to a sweet treat, rather than a regular component of one's everyday meals.

Please ensure to efficiently metabolize excess body fat.

The following principle primarily emphasizes the consumption of nutritious fats. Fats play a pivotal role in an individual's nutrition; however, it is important to emphasize the consumption of fats in their natural, unprocessed state. A proportion of these healthier fats can be found in natural food options such as nuts, seeds, avocados, and olive oil. Some animal-based food items that are high in beneficial fats include eggs, as well as oily fish such as salmon, mackerel, herring, and sardines. Incorporating extra virgin olive oil, avocado oil, or even coconut oil as a means of garnishing raw dishes such as salads, or for use during the process of cooking would be advantageous. Please be advised that in this particular dietary plan, it is permissible to consume animal and saturated fats derived from unprocessed sources, including but not limited to meats, fish, eggs, as well as butter or ghee. It is important to observe, however, that the consumption of saturated fat, particularly when combined with refined sugars and carbohydrates, can have detrimental effects on one's health. Furthermore, it is worth mentioning that commonly used oils such as vegetable, bean, and seed oils are often subjected to extensive processing and, as a result, are not recommended for consumption.

Consume Meat in Moderation

A remarkable aspect of the pegan diet is its allowance for the consumption of meat, even though it deviates significantly from traditional vegetarian dietary practices. In any event, irrespective of the permissibility of consuming meat, it is directed that its consumption during a meal should be restricted, serving more as a supplementary component or condiment, while vegetables should constitute the primary portion of the meal. Please be aware that aside from poultry or grass-fed meat, there are some alternative sources of animal protein that can be consumed, such as insects. However, this option may primarily appeal to those who possess a more adventurous spirit.

Consume whole grains and legumes.

Please ensure to only include whole grains in your diet while disregarding alternative types of grains. Indubitably, it is advised to abstain from the consumption of flours derived from grains. However, when it comes to whole grains, they should still be limited to small portions, typically no more than one cup per meal. Although it is true that some grains can possess high protein content, the primary focus should still be directed towards leafy vegetables. Beans are an excellent addition; however, it is advisable to refrain from using bland beans. Regardless, lentils and other similar legumes are highly beneficial for one's health, as they are excellent sources of fiber, protein, and minerals in one's diet. However, it is crucial to ensure that they are cooked thoroughly for proper consumption.

to limit the potential impacts of assimilation issues that may arise as a result of the consumption of beans.

Avoid handled sugars

Although it is not necessary to completely eliminate sugar from one's diet, it is advisable to minimize the consumption of refined sugars. The pegan diet aims to discourage the intake of substances that could potentially trigger insulin production and elevate blood sugar levels. Nevertheless, this does not imply that indulgence in sweet foods is strictly forbidden. However, it is strongly advised to exercise stringent control over their consumption, treating them as occasional indulgences rather than regular components of one's diet.

Limit Dairy Consumption

An aspect that many individuals who adhere to the vegetarian or paleo diet often find lacking is dairy. Dairy products are highly cherished across the globe, and the restriction of these items in paleo and vegan diets is a challenge that many individuals find difficult to overcome. In the context of this situation, dairy is deemed permissible within the framework of the pegan diet. However, due to the substantial impact dairy production has on the environment as a result of its manufacturing process, it is recommended that it be consumed in moderate quantities and, whenever possible, sourced from sustainable origins. Nevertheless, dairy can be regarded as a respectable source of protein.

Steer clear of artificial compounds and additives

To the greatest extent conceivable, it is advisable to refrain from the usage of synthetic compounds and additives in food products. This includes compound additives, preservatives, colorants, artificial sweeteners, or other undesirable ingredients. Genetically modified food sources are acceptable; however, it is preferable to prioritize natural food varieties to the greatest extent possible. Nevertheless, in light of the fact that genetically modified organisms (GMO) in food have been designed to enhance productivity by increasing food production per unit of land utilized, they also contribute to the advancement of sustainability. However, it is important to note that GMO food undergoes extensive processing, which necessitates their consumption in moderation.

Choose Sustainably Produced Foods

To the fullest extent possible, the consumption of food should primarily consist of sustainably produced food, driven not only by personal well-being but also by the imperative of preserving the planet and its ecosystems. To the utmost feasible extent, it is advisable to make use of natural, organically cultivated, and pasture-raised meats. When it comes to seafood, preference should be given to wild-caught varieties.

Fish is considered the optimal choice primarily because it consistently exhibits significantly lower levels of harmful substances, such as mercury,

100% of the time. However, it is imperative to ensure that the fish has been responsibly sourced to maintain sustainability.

What are the aspects that make the Pegan diet more intricate when compared to the Paleo and Vegan diets?

As previously discussed, the pegan diet combines elements from both the paleo and vegetarian diets, with the aim of incorporating as many benefits as possible while minimizing drawbacks. In this article, we examine the benefits and drawbacks of the paleo and vegetarian diets, and we explore how these are harmonized through the adoption of the pegan diet.

The Pros and Cons of Paleo and Vegan Diets, and How the Pegan Diet Addresses the Concerns Associated with the Vegan Diet, Including Weight Loss.

One of the primary motivations for individuals adopting a vegetarian diet is their pursuit of weight management. In light of the current global scenario, a significant number of individuals have attained excess weight as a result of overconsumption.

- the act of consuming excessive amounts of high-calorie food, including fast food and unhealthy snacks, which are rich in oils and sugars, particularly high-fructose corn syrup. Given the circumstances, people have begun to adopt vegetarian diets as a nutritious and low-calorie alternative to the prevalent and convenient fast food or frozen food trends. Taking all factors into consideration, it is logically sound to posit that a vegetarian diet facilitates weight loss, as the fundamental principle of losing weight rests on the premise that the calories expended should surpass the calorie intake. The most straightforward approach to achieving this objective is by decreasing the caloric intake of an individual. Vegetables and plant-based food options generally exhibit a significant reduction in caloric content compared to meats and other animal products. This signifies that, for an equivalent quantity of food consumed, individuals following a vegetarian diet intake considerably fewer calories when compared to those adhering to an omnivorous or carnivorous diet.

This hypothesis is substantiated in practical terms. Several scientific studies, which have been published in highly regarded academic journals like Nature and the American Journal of Clinical Nutrition, have drawn the conclusion that individuals who adhere to a vegan diet tend to exhibit lower body mass indexes. Various studies have indicated that individuals seeking to lose weight tend to experience faster weight loss when adhering to a vegetarian dietary approach. It is important to acknowledge that although it is typically ascribed to additional attributes, such as a more vigorous way of life, these investigations account for these supplementary influences, and ultimately affirm that vegan diets are associated with more pronounced weight reduction.

One remarkable aspect of this situation is that individuals following vegetarian diets are not necessarily subjected to feelings of restriction, as they are generally permitted to consume food until they feel satisfactorily full. This is the establishment that offers a selection of low-calorie and high

The inherent fibrous composition of most vegetarian diets results in a reduction of body weight, as it indicates that fewer calories are typically absorbed despite consuming a large quantity of food. The equivalent volume

The consumption of approximately 700 calories (700 kCal) from meat could potentially be reduced to a mere 200 calories (kCal) when consuming an equivalent volume of plant-based matter.

Improved Nutrition

In addition to facilitating weight loss, a remarkable aspect of adhering to a vegetarian diet is the fact that, ultimately, it tends to promote improved overall well-being. It is important to note that body weight and body mass index are not the sole, nor necessarily the most accurate, indicators of an individual's state of health. Nonetheless, while it may not be readily apparent, optimal nourishment can arguably be considered the most efficacious means of maintaining one's overall well-being and physical fitness. A person's external appearance may not necessarily reflect their true state of health and well-being; one can be unwell and lacking vitality despite not displaying any noticeable signs. This assertion suggests that the measurement of wellbeing should not solely rely on body weight.

Why would one prioritize enhancing their well-being over that of their counterparts? This outcome directly stems from the improved nourishment provided by their dietary choices. The abundance of nutrients found in vegetables, including but not limited to potassium, magnesium, Vitamins C and E, serves to ensure the body is adequately nourished to maintain its overall well-being and robustness. Despite the fact that vegetables are significantly richer in unsaturated fats (the beneficial type), along with their inherent abundance of dietary fiber and low cholesterol content, it follows that the consumption of vegetables tends to be significantly more advantageous for the body. This is primarily due to the reduced burden on the body's digestive processes when processing vegetable-based foods.

It is crucial to acknowledge, nonetheless, that vegetables inherently possess a multitude of vital nutrients, sufficiently meeting the body's requirements in those particular nutrients. Nonetheless, certain nutrients, such as Vitamin B-12, vitamin D, calcium, and specific fatty acids including the long-chain Omega-3 fatty acid found predominantly in fish, cannot be obtained through an exclusively plant-based diet. These nutrients cannot be synthesized by the body and thus must be obtained from an external source. The most optimal way for humans to acquire these nutrients is through the consumption of animal products, as they provide the most bio-available source. Therefore, vegetarians are advised to bolster their diet through appropriate supplementation, in order to ensure the acquisition of all necessary nutrients to maintain their overall well-being and uphold a balanced dietary intake.

Therefore, a vegetarian diet offers numerous health benefits, such as enhanced nutrition, given that vegetables and fruits inherently contain high levels of essential nutrients. However, it is important to note that while plants provide many nutrients, they do not supply all the essential ones. Therefore, it is necessary to supplement one's diet with appropriate nutritional supplements.

Reduced susceptibility to specific diseases

Individuals following a vegetarian diet employ a two-pronged approach to mitigate the risks associated with type-2 diabetes. First and foremost, it is worth mentioning that individuals frequently experience weight loss and successfully maintain it, which serves as an incredibly effective approach to assist the body in regulating elevated glucose levels. Secondly, their dietary pattern, which is predicated on plant-based consumption

In any instance, it is observable that fruits tend to reduce glucose levels due to their lower sugar content, as well as their substantial dietary fiber. Indeed, it has been demonstrated that, on the whole, individuals who adhere to a vegetarian diet have an approximate seventy

- There is a significant reduction in the risk of developing type-2 diabetes, with a decrease of eight percent (78%) noted. Moreover, individuals following a vegetarian diet have been observed to experience a glucose level that is up to two point four (2.4) times lower compared to other diets, as recommended by both the American Diabetes Association and the American Heart Association.

The benefits of adopting a vegetarian diet in reducing an individual's risk for disease are not confined solely to type-2 diabetes, but also extend to one of the most prevalent causes of death worldwide: cardiovascular disease. Numerous examinations have indicated that vegetarians frequently exhibit a reduction of approximately 75% in developing hypertension or high blood pressure, a risk factor for cardiovascular disease, as well as an overall decrease of 42% in the likelihood of dying from heart disease compared to the general population. Furthermore, there exist various illnesses for which the risks are diminished among individuals adhering to a vegetarian dietary regimen. One example pertains to the condition of cancer, wherein there exists a substantial decrease amounting to fifteen percent (15%) in the overall risk associated with the occurrence of any type of malignant growth. This significant reduction in risk can be attributed to the consistent maintenance of a vegetarian dietary regimen. Another ailment that poses a reduced risk for individuals who adhere to a vegetarian diet is renal disease. Vegans and vegetarians exhibited enhanced renal functions, characterized by an elevation in their glomerular filtration rate (GFR) and a decreased presence of creatinine and urea. These findings indicate that their kidneys are functioning optimally and experiencing a reduced workload in terms of filtration, when compared to individuals in other dietary categories.

that rely significantly on animal-based protein as a key component of their dietary intake.

Several distinct ailments that exhibit a reduced risk factor include Alzheimer's disease, a progressive neurodegenerative disorder characterized by cognitive decline, dementia, and ultimately mortality due to associated complications. Research has indicated an inclination towards a diminished prevalence (fewer occurrences) of Alzheimer's disease in individuals adhering to a vegetarian diet, while considering age and genetic factors as control variables. In addition to reducing the risk of Alzheimer's disease, a vegetarian diet has been observed to often result in a delayed onset of dementia among individuals diagnosed with Alzheimer's disease. This implies that vegetarians with Alzheimer's disease tend to maintain their cognitive faculties for a longer duration compared to the average patient.

A plant-based dietary regimen has also been demonstrated to contribute to the mitigation of certain manifestations of arthritis, including diminishing joint inflammation, alleviating a substantial degree of arthritic pain, and ameliorating the typical morning stiffness experienced by individuals with arthritis upon awakening.

The Advantages Of The Pegan Diet For Improving Health

Many individuals who have adhered to the Pegan diet have reported a multitude of additional health benefits in addition to achieving weight loss or weight management. Several additional medical benefits have been observed, including:

Reduced likelihood of developing cardiovascular disease.

One significant benefit of adopting a nutritious dietary plan is the promotion of cardiovascular well-being. Individuals who adhere to a dietary pattern characterized by rich inclusion of fresh fruits and vegetables, whole grains, vegetables, nuts, seeds, and lean proteins appear to exhibit a significantly reduced likelihood of experiencing cardiovascular ailments, including heart failure, stroke, and hypertension.

Lowers blood glucose levels.

Multiple studies have indicated that adhering to a well-balanced, customized meal plan can effectively mitigate the chances of developing diabetes and managing elevated blood sugar levels. In certain cases, it can even lead to the reversal of diabetes, including type 2 diabetes, without the reliance on daily medication.

Reduced Susceptibility to Alzheimer's Disease.

Owing to the abundant array of antioxidant properties, a nutritious diet comprising an abundance of fresh fruits and vegetables has been consistently demonstrated. The individual's susceptibility to developing Alzheimer's disease and other neuropsychiatric disorders is reduced.

Weight Reduction

Imposing limitations on unhealthy food options (processed, sugary, or foods high in unhealthy fats) has been shown to yield favorable outcomes for an individual's body composition. It frequently demonstrates that individuals who adhere to a healthy, balanced, and nutritious diet can achieve faster fat loss while preserving muscle mass, and sustain this weight loss over extended periods of time compared to their counterparts who do not.

Chapter Five:

Pegan Reference Guide

An introductory guide outlining the dietary requirements.

Consume a substantial amount

Non-dull vegetables

Organic produce with a low glycemic index (such as berries, kiwis, oranges, etc.)

Eggs

Fish with low mercury levels, such as salmon, mackerel, sardines, anchovies, and similar varieties.

Consume a reasonable quantity.

Low-glycemic grains, such as black rice or quinoa (with a portion size of up to ½ cup per meal)

An appropriate daily intake of both beans and vegetables would be limited to a maximum of one cup.

Organically-raised, pasture-fed meat and poultry (serving size ranging from 4 to 6 ounces per meal)

Nutritious fats (such as olive oil, avocado oil, coconut oil, clarified butter, plant-based spreads)

Consume a morsel.

Bland vegetables

Natural products that have a high glycemic index, such as grapes, melons, cherries, and similar fruits

Edible kernels and grains

Dairy products derived from goat or sheep's milk.

Infrequent Treats

Dehydrated organic goods

Juices

Sugar

Alcoholic beverages (limited to a maximum of 2 servings per week)

Maintain distance from" or "Avoid

Managed the procurement and storage of food supplies

Dairy products derived from cow's milk (excluding incidental substances such as margarine or ghee)

Various types of vegetable oils including canola, corn, soybean, sunflower, and others

Recommended Food Resources for Inclusion in the Pegan Diet

The primary dietary component of the Pegan diet consists of vegetables and organic produce, which should account for 75% of your total consumption.

It is important to emphasize the consumption of low-glycemic fruits and vegetables such as berries and non-starchy vegetables in order to mitigate the impact on blood glucose levels. Individuals who have already achieved stable glucose control prior to commencing the diet may wish to consider incorporating a restricted amount of insipid vegetables and naturally sweetened organic produce into their regimen. Individuals adhering to the Pegan diet are encouraged to consume meals that prioritize the inclusion of unprocessed whole food sources, meaning food sources that have undergone minimal processing and retain their natural structure prior to being brought into an individual's kitchen.

Non-Starchy Vegetables

Mixed Greens

Cauliflower

Broccoli

Brussel Sprouts

Celery

Spinach

Asparagus

New Fruit

Bananas

Berries

Apples

Peaches

Pears

Apri-beds

Cherries

Grapes

Melon

Capably Sourced Proteins

Skinless Pigeon Breast

Reduced-Fat Beef Selections

Pork

Seafood

Eggs

Skinless Turkey

Tempeh

Wild Salmon

Sardines

Solid Fats

The list includes avocados, olives, copra oil, olive oil, and avocado oil.

Nuts and Seeds

The assortment comprises of various types of nutritious seeds and nuts such as almonds, walnuts, flaxseed, chia seed, hemp seeds, and pistachios.

Vegetables

Black beans, lentils, kidney beans, garbanzo beans.

Grains

Dusky Rice, Millet, Oats, Quinoa.

The Pantry with a Blend of Paleo and Vegan Delicacies

Simplify the process of food preparation by stocking your pantry with these well-documented food sources that adhere to the Pegan diet.

Vegetables

Beets

Broccoli

Brussels sprouts

Leeks

Onions

Garlic

Ginger
Bok choy
Squash
Cauliflower
Tomatoes
Spinach
Green beans
Kale
Chard
Peppers
Cucumbers
Turnips
Yams
Carrots
Radishes
Asparagus

Organic Products
Bananas
Oranges
Grapefruit
Organic product made with Kiwi
Pears
Nectarines
Blueberries

Raspberries
Strawberries
Avocados
Lemons
Limes
Protein
Eggs
Organic, pasture-raised meat.
Low-mercury fish
Tofu
Tempeh
Edamame
Solid Fats
Olive oil
Avocado oil
Coconut oil
Ghee
Nuts
Seeds
Starches
Dark rice
Red rice
Quinoa
Soba noodles
Beans

Lentils

Dairy
Authentic, herbaceous-maintained spread made from plant oil
Ghee
Yogurt
Kefir
Goat's cheddar
Various
Vinegar
New spices
Stock
Tahini
Almond milk
Coconut milk
Enhancements
Nutrient D
Nutrient B12
Desserts
Nectar
Maple syrup
Dim chocolate
Foods to Exclude from the Pegan Diet's Assortment

The Pegan diet exhibits greater flexibility compared to both paleo and vegetarian diets as it allows for spontaneous consumption of nearly all types of food.

Taking all factors into account, certain food varieties and nutritional categories are undeniably weakened. Certain food options can be deemed less desirable, while others can be considered highly nutritious, depending on the perspective of the individual being asked.

The Pegan diet consistently excludes the consumption of these food sources:

• Dairy products such as cow's milk, yogurt, and cheddar cheese are considerably weakened. However, it should be noted that limited quantities of food products derived from sheep or goat milk are permitted. Occasionally, the application of grass control measures is also authorized.

• Gluten: All grains that contain gluten are unquestionably incapacitating.

• Gluten-free grains: Even grains devoid of gluten are weakened. Occasional allowances may be made for small amounts of gluten-free whole grains.

• Legumes: The majority of vegetables are weakened as a result of their ability to generate glucose. Lentils, which are classified as low-starch vegetables, could potentially be considered permissible.

• Sugar: It is generally avoided to include any form of added sugar, whether refined or unrefined. Alright, it may be employed on occasion, albeit in limited measure.

• Processed oils: Oils that have undergone extensive refining or processing, such as canola, soybean, sunflower, and vegetable oil, are frequently avoided.

• Food additives: Artificial dyes, flavorings, additives, and other substances are to be avoided.

A significant proportion of these food sources is restricted owing to their evident impact on glucose or potential exacerbation in the body.

Introduction

The Pegan diet is an innovative and contemporary dietary approach, drawing inspiration from the well-established and widely recognized dietary trends of paleo and veganism.

The Pegan diet integrates the fundamental benefits of both, considering their principal components and concepts. Consequently, it is purported to possess greater health benefits in comparison to both of those dietary regimens. However, it is important to not be deceived by its title as this dietary regimen does not adhere to vegan principles. There exist valid justifications for this deviation, which shall be elaborated upon in subsequent discussion.

In conclusion, adherents of the paleo diet strive to consume foods that were prevalent approximately 2.6 million years ago, during the Paleolithic period, including vegetables, fruits, nuts, meat, and fish. Paleo adherents abstain from incorporating processed foods, sodium and sucrose, cereals and pulses, dairy-derived oils, sodium, and naturally, caffeinated beverages and alcoholic beverages, into their dietary regimen.

In contrast, individuals who adhere to a vegan lifestyle solely consume meals derived from plants and refrain from consuming any animal-derived products, including but not limited to meat, fish, and their byproducts.

Products such as eggs, dairy, or honey. In contrast to individuals who adhere to a paleo diet, they consume grains, beans, and other legumes, in addition to plant-based fats and oils.

The Pegan diet improves overall physical well-being by decreasing inflammation, regulating blood glucose levels, and providing ample energy to the body.

This objective can be achieved through the abundant consumption of fresh vegetables, fruits, and whole foods, alongside the moderation of meat, fish, and dairy product intake. The Pegan diet is designed to be embraced as a long-term lifestyle choice as opposed to a short-term weight loss solution. It promotes a daily commitment to mindful eating. Each year, an increasing number of individuals opt to experience it, driven by its advantageous impact on one's health.

If one takes pleasure in partaking of an assorted array of fruits and vegetables, yet occasionally experiences a yearning for meat or fish, this dietary regimen may prove to be well-suited.

7

BENEFITS AND DOWNSIDES

The Pegan diet underscores the consumption of nutritious and unprocessed meals that are abundant in essential vitamins and minerals, thereby offering several health advantages for your well-being. It is also fundamentally simple and uncomplicated. In contrast to alternative dietary approaches, there is no necessity to quantify the quantities of proteins, carbohydrates, or calories, thereby facilitating straightforward long-term monitoring.

The adherence to the Pegan diet may lead to substantial weight reduction, as it necessitates the elimination of detrimental food sources such as those high in starch and sugar, contingent upon one's present dietary habits. Furthermore, the dietary plan places emphasis on the consumption of nutrient-rich foods that contribute to the enhancement of various aspects of overall well-being, in addition to facilitating weight loss.

The Pegan diet predominantly consists of fruits and vegetables, renowned for their abundant nutrient content, including fiber, minerals, and vitamins. This will supply your body with vital energy, fortify your immune system, and enhance the overall condition of your skin and hair.

8

The Pegan diet promotes the consumption of nutrient-rich fats derived from sources such as fish, nuts, seeds, and plant-based products, while advising against the intake of unhealthy fats and processed foods. Consuming unfavorable fats, specifically omega-6 fatty acids, can lead to detrimental health effects such as elevated cholesterol levels, persistent inflammation, and the development of cardiovascular disease. In contrast, consumption of nutrient-rich fats such as omega-3 fatty acids exerts a favorable effect on the body, devoid of any adverse consequences. Moreover, it enhances the levels of beneficial cholesterol in the bloodstream and facilitates the assimilation of essential vitamins A, K, and other vitamins that are soluble in fats.

By refraining from consuming processed foods, you will establish a safeguard against incorporating any synthetic pigments, enhancers, additives, or other constituents, as well as excessive quantities of sweeteners or sodium, all of which possess the potential to be detrimental to your well-being.

When the Pegan diet is adhered to in a correct and diligent manner, it can be deemed safe and is generally not accompanied by any notable adverse effects. Nevertheless, it is imperative that you take into consideration the subsequent apprehensions.

9

The primary and utmost consideration is consistently centered on your present state of health. Prior to making any substantial modifications to your current dietary regimen, it is advisable to engage in a conversation with your healthcare provider or a qualified nutritionist, especially if you have any preexisting medical conditions of concern.

This dietary regimen may pose challenges for individuals adhering to a vegan or vegetarian lifestyle due to its incorporation of animal-derived ingredients. The Pegan diet imposes limitations on the daily intake of whole grains and legumes, which are the fundamental components of a plant-centric diet. In contrast, meat offers essential minerals like iron, vitamin B12, calcium, and potassium that are comparatively challenging to acquire through a vegan dietary approach.

Adhering solely to a vegan adaptation of the Pegan diet could present challenges, necessitating careful attention to ensure an adequate intake of protein and other essential nutrients on a daily basis. It is highly recommended that you strictly conform to all the guiding principles of the Pegan diet, rather than focusing solely on its vegan component.

The Pegan diet may pose a challenge for individuals who consume meat. Due to the absence of other food groups, individuals may consume excessive amounts of it. Prolonged adherence to a diet characterized by elevated protein levels and minimal carbohydrate consumption has the potential to lead to kidney complications and osteoporosis among certain individuals.

10

Additionally, it is crucial to emphasize that the Pegan diet restricts consumption of a diverse range of foods that are traditionally considered nourishing and advantageous for individual well-being. Legumes, such as are an exemplary source of protein, fiber, and minerals such as iron, zinc, and copper. A similar rationale applies to wholegrains, as they serve as an extremely nutritious resource that has the potential to contribute to the prevention of various chronic health conditions. As an illustration, the consumption of animal milk has the capacity to furnish one's body with essential minerals like calcium, vitamin D, protein, and potassium.

Nonetheless, it is typically proscribed within the confines of the Pegan diet. Accordingly, several experts recommend that individuals following a pagan diet occasionally consume a limited quantity of foods and food groups that are typically restricted, in order to maintain a balanced and equitable assortment of nutrients.

In addition, this diet emphasizes a plethora of fresh ingredients and animal products that are obtained through sustainable sourcing methods. Although these food options are undeniably beneficial for your well-being in the long term, they typically come with a higher price tag and may have a financial impact.

However, should you adhere to the dietary guidelines meticulously, meticulously plan your meals in advance, and ensure sufficient intake of nutrient-rich and varied foods, it is highly likely that you will experience no adverse effects. Following an extended duration on the Pegan diet, individuals will experience increased vitality and a sense of lightness. The enhancement of skin and hair radiance can be attributed to the plentiful supply of essential vitamins and minerals. Additionally, weight loss will occur and overall physical well-being will be positively impacted.

Cheesy Muffins

Ingredients

- ¼ cup almond meal 1/8

- cup flax seeds meal

- Salt, to taste

- ¼ cup low-fat cottage cheese

- ¼ cup scallion, sliced thinly

- ¼ cup raw hemp seeds

- ¼ teaspoon baking powder

- 1/8 cup nutritional yeast flakes

- ¼ cup Parmesan cheese, grated finely

- 3 organic eggs, beaten

Directions

1. Set the broiler to a temperature of 360 degrees Fahrenheit and lightly grease two biscuit cups with oil.

2. Incorporate almond feast, flax seeds, hemp seeds, baking powder, and salt in a mixing bowl, ensuring thorough integration.

3. Combine cottage cheese, Parmesan cheese, nutritional yeast flakes, and egg in a separate bowl.

4. Integrate the mixture of cheddar and almond together and blend until thoroughly amalgamated.

5. Incorporate the scallions and transfer this mixture into the greased biscuit cups.

6. Move the mixture into the oven and commence the preparation process for approximately 30 minutes.

7. To promptly serve or prepare for an evening meal, you may opt to refrigerate the biscuits in the refrigerator for a duration of 3-4 days. Please ensure they are adequately covered with a paper towel and subsequently reheated prior to usage.

Cauliflower Gnocchi Prepared With A Minimalistic Approach

Ingredients:
For the gnocchi:

Cassava flour, ¾ cup
Minced cauliflower, 4 cups

Sea salt, ½ teaspoon

For the sauce:

Large garlic cloves, 2 pieces
Tapioca flour, 2 tablespoons
Salt and pepper

Full-fat canned coconut milk, 4 cups
Spinach, 4 cups

Instructions:

1. Commence by preheating the oven to a temperature of 425 degrees Fahrenheit. Next, steam the cauliflower separately until it reaches a tender consistency. Remove the water by using an absorbent towel and wring out any remaining moisture.

Combine the active components for the gnocchi in a mixer until achieving a silky consistency; incorporate the cassava flour in an amount adequate enough to allow the dough to be easily kneaded.

Proceed to divide the dough into four equal portions and shape them into cylinders measuring approximately 3/4 inches in diameter. After completion, divide the tubes into pieces measuring one inch in length.

Bring water to a boil in a large skillet and add the gnocchi, reducing the heat. Once they have ascended to the uppermost layer, delicately extract and generously distribute a modest amount of olive oil onto them.

To begin, procure a cooking tray and proceed to line it with parchment paper. Proceed by drizzling a small amount of olive oil evenly over the parchment paper on the tray. Once the 20-minute timeframe has elapsed, proceed to flip the gnocchi and continue baking it for an additional 20 minutes.

With regards to the sauce, incorporate all the ingredients, excluding the spinach, into a saucepan and vigorously whisk them throughout the process. Furthermore, you have the option to utilize a handheld immersion blender. Continue performing the said action until the sauce begins to achieve a denser consistency. Consistent agitation will undoubtedly inhibit the formation of lumps in the sauce. Please incorporate spinach at a later stage and blend it with the gnocchi.

Advantages Of The Pagan Diet

In addition to the aforementioned advantages of the Pegan diet, which include its positive impact on the environment and incorporation of beneficial aspects from both the Vegan and Paleo diets, there exist numerous reasons to consider adopting the Pegan diet as a means of pursuing a healthy lifestyle. Adhering to the principles of the Pegan diet, particularly for those new to it, yields optimal advantages.

A significant advantage of the Pegan diet lies in its wide accessibility to the majority of individuals, while remaining fairly economical. The Pegan diet does not necessitate any specialized training or significant investment of time to adhere to its principles. If one should consider anything, it would be the fact that the cost of Pegan diet meal plans is notably more affordable in comparison to the majority of standard meals. This is due to the fact that fruits and vegetables, exemplifying a significant portion of the Pegan diet, are more economically feasible compared to the majority of meal options.

Pegan diet meals do not necessitate extensive culinary skills due to their reduced reliance on cooking techniques. Minimal dedication to your schedule is also required. There is no need for you to allocate time towards the amalgamation of vegetables and fruits; it is likely that you will solely need to engage in the process of steaming or boiling your protein sources, which should not impose a significant time constraint, incidentally. It is crucial to note that one should primarily refrain from consuming processed seasonings rather than organic alternatives when adhering to the Pegan diet.

Replace seasoning cubes and other highly processed seasonings with natural alternatives such as garlic, ginger, mint leaves, and turmeric. Essentially, the Pegan diet promotes dietary flexibility, offers a cost-effective approach, and is highly feasible to adhere to. Indeed, it can be confidently asserted that the Pegan diet represents a viable solution to a lengthy history of unsuccessful dietary approaches characterized by excessive limitations, high costs, or intricate maintenance requirements. As a novice adherent of the Pegan diet, although adhering to a dietary regimen may pose some challenges, the Pegan diet facilitates the adoption of a wholesome lifestyle through its associated dietary principles. The Pegan diet is known to induce a significant lifestyle transformation that often yields consequences across various facets of one's life. The Pegan diet has a documented track record of enduring efficacy, and the advantages persist even amidst minor modifications to the dietary regimen. This outcome can be attributed to the absence of dairy products in the Pegan diet, as substantiated by scientific evidence from nutritionists and dieticians, which establishes that dairy foods contribute to the occurrence of health conditions such as asthma and eczema. According to nutrition and diet experts, dairy products are known to induce inflammation in the body and foster an environment that is favorable for the development of autoimmune disorders. Therefore, it follows that particular dairy products, particularly those derived from animals that are not fed on pasture, have the potential to facilitate the development of conditions such as asthma and other respiratory ailments by producing a conducive environment for the occurrence of such diseases. Individuals exhibiting symptoms of these diseases are typically counseled to incorporate Pegan diet meal plans into their overall dietary regimen, with the aim of excluding dairy products from their food intake. The exclusion of dairy products within the Pegan diet additionally enhances vitality, fortifies the immune system, and facilitates the detoxification process within the body.

The Pegan diet is predominantly plant-based, with approximately three-quarters of the diet being vegan and one-quarter adhering to the principles of the paleo diet. Consequently, the proportion of proteins is significantly lower compared to vegetables. One benefit of this is that extensive research conducted over the course of several years has demonstrated that a significant intake of meat, particularly those sourced from non-locally grown animals raised with growth-enhancing chemicals, culminates in various adverse outcomes. While protein intake may be crucial for growth, particularly among individuals in their formative years, augmenting consumption could heighten susceptibility to ailments such as arthritis, particularly as individuals advance in age. Excessive protein intake has the potential to contribute to the emergence of cardiovascular ailments and diminished cardiac well-being. By adhering to the Pegan diet, which restricts protein intake, particularly from meat, the likelihood of developing cardiovascular conditions is significantly diminished.

Additionally, it should be noted that fruits and vegetables, being the cornerstone of the Pegan diet, exhibit a remarkable range of nutritional diversity. Fruits and vegetables possess abundant dietary fiber, vitamins, minerals, and phytochemicals which are acknowledged for their disease-preventive effects and ability to mitigate oxidative stress and inflammation. The Pegan diet also incorporates nutritious and monounsaturated fats sourced from fish, nuts, seeds, and other plant-based foods, which contribute to the enhancement of cardiovascular health. The Pegan diet is additionally centered around the consumption of whole foods, leading to an enhanced dietary profile and ultimately, an improvement in individual well-being.

It should be noted that the Pegan diet combines elements from the Paleo diet and the Vegan diet, incorporating advantageous aspects from both regimes to enhance the overall benefits of the Pegan diet. The Paleo diet often receives reproach for its disregard towards environmental concerns, as it depletes the earth's natural resources and contributes to air pollution and excessive water consumption. The Pegan diet mitigates potential harm to the environment and optimizes resource utilization by promoting the procurement and consumption of sustainably produced food and meat, thereby reducing ecological risks.

For individuals desiring to adopt a proper dietary regimen, with the aim of starting any form of dietary plan, the Pegan diet is highly recommended due to its long-term viability. This can be attributed to the fact that the Pegan diet establishes a balanced and holistic approach that bridges the gap between the Vegan and Paleo diets. Both the Vegan and the Paleo diets exhibit considerable restrictions and present challenges in terms of adherence, thus the Pegan diet strives to engender a state of equilibrium while permitting a certain degree of adaptability.

Primary Advantages Of The Pegan Diet

1. "The focal point of the diet and its most significant nutritional advantage lies in the emphasis placed on consuming fruits and vegetables." Vegetables and fruits possess a bounty of essential vitamins, minerals, phytochemicals, and dietary fiber, rendering them highly nutritious. Consumption of these natural products aids in averting the advent of ailments and mitigating inflammation in the body.

2. The pagan diet places emphasis on the ingestion of nourishing fats sourced from whole foods such as fish caught in the wild, various nuts and seeds, avocados, and olives, which

have also been associated with enhancing cardiovascular well-being.

3. Decreasing the consumption of processed food items that are laden with a variety of artificial sweeteners and chemical additives assists in augmenting the nutritional variety and richness of one's diet. It mitigates adverse impacts arising from the presence of additives, pesticides, and chemicals.

4. The pagan diet advocates for the consumption of nutrient-dense and unprocessed foods, which are abundant in a wide array of essential vitamins and minerals crucial for maintaining optimal bodily functions. Based on the assessment of your existing dietary habits, substantial weight loss through adherence to a pagan diet is anticipated.

5. In the case of individuals adhering to a conventional Western diet comprising heavily of processed foods, the potential effects of adopting the pagan diet might be more pronounced compared to those who already maintain a generally nutritious diet.

6. It is also comparatively easy to comprehend and adhere to. In contrast to alternative dietary approaches, the pegan diet does not necessitate the meticulous tracking of macros, points, calories, or carbohydrates, rendering it significantly more convenient to adhere to overall.

7. Furthermore, the dietary plan places significant emphasis on incorporating nutritious elements, thereby fostering improvements in various facets of individuals' well-

being apart from just weight reduction, such as cardiovascular wellness, glycemic control, and the prevention of ailments. The pegan diet encompasses a range of valuable elements that can be regarded as excellent supplements to a comprehensive and balanced diet. These elements include nutritious oils, assorted fruits and vegetables, a variety of the most nutritious nuts, seeds, and sustainable sources of protein.

The Significance Of Integrating Physical Exercise With Adherence To The Pegan Dietary Regimen

In the forthcoming chapter, our objective is to provide a comprehensive elucidation of how sports can prove immensely beneficial, both at fundamental and advanced stages, in attaining nutritional objectives. Furthermore, this holds particularly true in the context of a Pegan diet. As is the case with any dietary regimen, exercise represents the appropriate approach, if not the indispensable one. This is due to the fact that the dietary regimen typically necessitates a reduction in caloric intake, thereby creating a caloric deficit conducive to weight loss. By incorporating the calorie expenditure from physical activities into the calorie reduction accomplished through dietary changes, the likelihood of witnessing this outcome is further heightened. Furthermore, if we consider the incorporation of physical activity within the context of the Pegan diet, we will not only observe significant weight loss results but also experience one of the most profound advantages associated with this dietary approach. One of the primary advantages and characteristics of the Pegan diet lies in its fundamental objective, which is to achieve a genuine reorientation of one's dietary patterns in order to recalibrate the metabolism. With the integration of physical activity, this process can be further expedited and accomplished.

Nevertheless, exercise caution as it may not be essential, particularly in an authoritarian regime such as Pegan, that individuals possess a high level of athleticism. Due to this rationale, we have elected to delineate the Pegan diet as a protocol for fundamental athleticism within one paragraph, while allocating a separate paragraph for specific strategies and supplements geared towards individuals engaged in competitive sports.

Reverting to the Pegan diet and exercise discussion, we can reconvene with the aforementioned points and assert that this regimen necessitates concomitant participation in fundamental physical activity. This signifies, to be precise, that when discussing sports to complement the Pegan diet, we are referring to sports suitable for novice individuals. It is not necessary to possess the qualities of a marathon runner or be a professional in cross-fit in order to adhere to this dietary plan, as it is based on the assumption that an increased intake of macronutrients, particularly carbohydrates, is required.

With that being stated, the sport in question pertains to the one that is widely observed within domestic or park settings. Accordingly, it is a sport that exclusively focuses on the body's movement and serves the practical goal of weight reduction. Engaging in athletic activities that demand high levels of physical exertion, such as running or bodybuilding, can be perilous.

Regarding the latter point, it has been previously mentioned that the recommended exercise regimen to complement this dietary plan is bodyweight training, specifically excluding the use of weights. Nevertheless, individuals with a smaller build are permitted, but their presence should be kept to a minimum.

In any event, the integration of appropriate physical exercise becomes crucial within the context of the Pegan diet to attain enhanced outcomes. Our intention is not to enumerate all the advantages of regular physical activity, but rather to present those in conjunction with the Pegan diet:

• Initially, as previously mentioned, the combination of adhering to a Pegan diet and engaging in physical activity will effectively establish the requisite caloric deficit for expediting weight loss.

• It will facilitate an acceleration of your metabolism: as previously mentioned, the purpose of this diet is to provide our individuals with knowledge about proper nutrition and subsequently restore a sluggish metabolic rate. Incorporating regular physical activity will enhance the efficiency of your metabolic processes, thus ensuring sustainable outcomes.

• Incorporating physical activity into the Pegan lifestyle would result in greater enhancements in terms of improving health. When discussing conditions like cardiovascular disorders or diabetes, we reviewed how the Pegan diet plays a significant role in managing and averting these issues. Further support for this assertion lies in the fact that incorporating physical exercise will have a pronounced effect on insulin levels, blood glucose levels, and overall blood pressure regulation.

After elucidating the significance of integrating sport into the Pegan diet, we aim to furnish you with practical recommendations for its optimal implementation, catering firstly to individuals engaging in non-professional athletic pursuits, followed by guidelines tailored specifically for professionals.

Suggestions for individuals with limited athletic experience

We have previously stated that it is feasible to engage in bodyweight training in both residential and outdoor settings. We would like to emphasize that due to the consistently restrictive nature of this regimen, it is of utmost importance to exercise caution and refrain from excessively engaging in physical activities. By following this course of action, you would solely be exposed to the potentiality of physical debilitation.

In any event, presented below are several valuable suggestions for engaging in physical activity while adhering to a Pegan dietary regimen:

• Initially, prioritize engaging in cardio exercises with low impact. By this, we imply that engaging in physical activities that do not excessively strain one's respiratory or cardiovascular systems is the optimal choice for individuals adhering to a dietary regimen. In practical application, these activities primarily comprise of low-impact cardiovascular exercises such as brisk walking, utilizing stationary bicycles, or engaging in cycling on flat terrain. These activities also provide a moderate caloric expenditure, thereby supporting your dietary objectives without depleting your body's energy reserves.

• Exercise restraint: there is no obligation to engage in the activities on a daily basis. Performing cardiovascular exercise two to three times per week will suffice. Certainly, we have no intention of discouraging you from engaging in daily walks. Furthermore, aside from its tangible dietary benefits, walking proves advantageous not just for our physical well-being but also for our mental equilibrium.

• Please ensure that you do not exceed the designated training time of 1 hour; allowing 1 hour and a half for training will be sufficient. Engaging in further activities while adhering to a restrictive diet could pose a potential hazard.

• Should you choose to utilize weights, it is imperative to bear in mind the importance of refraining from the employment of an excessive load. Individuals of lesser strength who possess appropriate repetitions are acceptable.

• It is imperative to consistently engage in muscle relaxation exercises, as stretching holds significant importance in promoting muscle relaxation and facilitating their cooldown.

• In relation to the aforementioned, yoga presents itself as an optimal form of physical activity within the context of the Pegan diet, given its low demand for exertion while simultaneously enhancing both psychological and physical wellness.

The aforementioned recommendations represent the optimal guidelines pertaining to the fundamental physical activity linked to the Pegan dietary regimen. The primary principle is to exercise moderation and consistently seek guidance from medical professionals for personalized advice.

Guidelines for individuals seeking to enhance their competitiveness in sports.

In the previous paragraph, we have provided you with all the best tips regarding non-competitive sport and the Pegan diet.

Now, we shall proceed to discuss individuals who engage in sports at a competitive level. We have come to the determination to partition these two components due to their stark contrast in levels of difficulty. One initial challenge pertains to the very observation that an individual engaged in sport at a rudimentary level, lacking professional training, will inevitably not exert the same level of effort or maintain a similar frequency as those dedicated to professional training.

Previously, we provided counsel regarding the prudence of avoiding excessive physical activity in terms of frequency and duration if one is adhering to the Pegan dietary regimen. This can be attributed to the potential depletion of energy, leaving individuals ill-equipped to confront more substantial or sustained endeavors.

Consider even more if you find yourself confronted with the challenge of participating in a marathon or a specialized professional sports competition that necessitates specific preparatory measures and a heightened level of physical vitality.

Indeed, an additional level of complexity arises in relation to the elevated energy requirements associated with professional sports. Hence, adhering to the stringent principles of the Pegan regime and engaging in sports with greater intensity and continuity remains an illusory concept.

Nevertheless, we maintain that it is crucial to cultivate some form of logical thinking. As previously mentioned, sport and diet are two inseparable unions with strong practical implications. Engaging in physical exercise aids in achieving weight loss goals and enhances metabolic adjustment. Similarly, adopting an appropriate dietary regimen assists in optimizing physical fitness and enhancing professional performance during sports activities.

The divergence lies in the primary objective: within the realm of professional athletics, it is commonly believed that weight loss is not a requirement, hence the recommended dietary regimen only aims to enhance overall physical performance. Optimal physical condition, hence not necessarily synonymous with tangible weight reduction.

Nevertheless, if one still desires to adhere to a nutritious diet in order to enhance their athletic abilities, how does one proceed?

To begin, it is advisable to seek guidance from a medical nutritionist regarding the suitability, sustainability, and effectiveness of the aforementioned regimen, particularly if you are a professional athlete. Consulting with your physician will provide you with a comprehensive understanding of how such a dietary plan aligns with your individual requirements and goals.

However, it must be noted that should you choose to adopt this diet, it would be virtually impossible to adhere to its exceedingly stringent guidelines. This is attributed to the fact that an individual who engages in an extensive regimen of physical activity, as mentioned earlier, requires a substantial amount of energy. The primary source of energy that is recognized stems predominantly from carbohydrates. Hence, in this particular instance, opting for a low carbohydrate diet would not be the optimal decision. However, it is indeed feasible to modify the Pegan diet to cater to individuals engaged in competitive sports, provided they receive additional guidance and strategies.

As a result, in order to adhere to this specific dietary regimen, it is necessary to observe the following measures:

• Initially, it is advisable to augment the quantity of carbohydrates to be consumed in the dietary intake. Furthermore, it is imperative to incorporate an appropriate quantity of carbohydrates into your dietary regimen, alongside proteins and vegetables. It is imperative to consistently opt for whole grains, legumes, and all food items with known origins, while avoiding packaged snacks, industrial snacks, and refined flours.

• Augmenting serving sizes: rumors have surfaced regarding the potential amplification of portions in a broader context. This holds particularly true for individuals engaged in vigorous physical activities where an elevated intake of proteins and vitamins is imperative. Hence, it is imperative not only to incorporate carbohydrates into your Pegan diet but also to amplify the quantities of meat, fish, eggs, and vegetables.

• It is crucial not to overlook the consumption of organic fruit, as it serves as a vital source of immediate energy for athletic activities. It also boasts a high concentration of vital vitamins and nutrients.

These measures will prove advantageous should you desire to adhere to a nutritious dietary regimen while simultaneously retaining optimal physical and athletic well-being. Now, we conclude this chapter pertaining to the correlation between the Pegan diet and physical activity. In the subsequent chapter, we shall elucidate the practical aspects of this dietary regimen, delineating the permissible food choices and cautioning against the consumption of certain items.

Preparing To Go Pegan

The adoption of the Pegan diet is increasingly prevalent in contemporary times, representing a prevailing trend in the realm of dietary practices. Can you eat meat? Certainly, it is permissible to do so, provided that it is not done in an exaggerated manner.

What about processed ingredients? You are limited to consuming only a small quantity. This dietary plan primarily consists of whole foods, encompassing a variety of fresh vegetables and fruits that will be incorporated into your meals.

The Pegan diet amalgamates the principles of vegan and paleo diets, underpinned by the notion that the consumption of unprocessed, nutrient-dense foods promotes peak physical well-being through the amelioration of inflammation and stabilization of blood sugar levels.

At initial observation, the notion of amalgamating vegan and paleo diets may appear contradictory or unconventional. Nevertheless, you can be reassured that it is not. Alternatively, one should consider it as a harmonious amalgamation that combines the most advantageous aspects of both dietary approaches.

Fundamentally, meal planning is quite uncomplicated. As previously stated, the recipes of the Pegan diet incorporate limited quantities of premium animal-derived proteins, an abundance of nutritious fats, as well as a variety of fruits and vegetables. Moreover, it will be necessary for you to abstain from consuming legumes, including peanuts, lentils, peas, and beans, as well as grains and dairy products.

The principles underlying both the vegan and paleo diets encompass:

Employing fats of superior quality: fats derived from olive oil, seeds, nuts, avocados, and sources enriched with omega-3 fatty acids.

Minimal pesticide content: Consider opting for organic produce that is free from hormones, antibiotics, and genetically modified organisms (GMOs).

No chemical substances: Absence of substances such as MSG, synthetic colorings, artificial sweeteners, or any other synthetic additives.

Abundant selection of vegetables and fruits: Seek out shades that are rich and vibrant; the greater the assortment, the more desirable.

Low glycemic load: Devoid of processed carbohydrates, refined flour, and added sugars.

Upon selecting the Pegan diet as your dietary choice, you will:

Consume sugary products in moderation; indulge in them on occasions as a special indulgence.

Refrain from consuming legumes, grains, and dairy products.

It is advisable to incorporate a substantial amount of seeds and nuts into your diet, as they possess a high protein content and help mitigate the chances of developing diabetes and heart ailments.

Consume primarily vegetables, comprising approximately 75% of the daily dietary intake.

Incorporate beneficial fats into your diet, such as omega-3 fatty acids, seeds, olive oil, nuts, and avocados, while refraining from the consumption of soybean and vegetable oils.

Consume food with a reduced glycemic load; alternatively, opt for elevated levels of fats and proteins found in ingredients such as sardines, olive oil, seeds, nuts, and avocados.

Controversy

The surge in popularity of Pegan recipes and diet has been notable, starting from 2014. An illustrative example would be the substantial increase in searches for 'eating Pegan' on Pinterest, soaring to a remarkable 337% in 2021. Nevertheless, this dietary approach has not been without its controversies.

For instance, according to expert recommendations, the fundamental principles of this diet entail merging two contrasting diet ideologies to create a novel dietary approach. Nevertheless, in actuality, they maintain the viewpoint that the majority of the limitations imposed by a Pegan diet are burdensome in terms of time, expense, and lack practicality.

An issue could arise with regard to restricting legumes, as pointed out by these authorities in the field of nutrition and diet. In accordance with research findings, legumes have been determined to be low in fat, abundant in dietary fiber, and a significant protein source that constitutes an essential component of the widely acclaimed Mediterranean dietary pattern. Furthermore, there is evidence suggesting that legumes are associated with various health advantages such as the mitigation of cardiovascular ailments, cancer, and more.

Positive Reports

Although there have been instances of controversy surrounding the Pegan diet, it has also garnered numerous favorable responses. It is widely recognized by experts that supporting local produce and prioritizing freshness is highly favorable. Additionally, the majority of these experts concur with Dr. Hyman's perspective that animal-based products should be regarded as supplementary rather than fundamental items in one's diet. Furthermore, researchers also hold a fondness for the notion of augmenting the consumption of vegetables, fruits, and seafood.

Consensus has been reached among others regarding the multiple dimensions of a Pegan diet. Notably, this dietary approach offers significant benefits such as a focus on important nutrients like omega-3 fatty acids, as well as an emphasis on the consumption of fruits and vegetables. Furthermore, another notable factor contributing to the advantages of this diet is the provision of appropriate protein intake. In essence, it can be argued that adopting a Pegan diet may yield significant benefits for one's physical well-being. Nevertheless, there are certain limitations that you must adhere to. Should you possess the capacity to do so, implementing the Pegan diet will commence yielding favorable outcomes for your physical well-being.

The Pegan Shopping List

Now that you are aware of the requirements, we present to you a selection of essential products that should undeniably find a place on your shopping itinerary:

Vegetables: It is important to incorporate vegetables into your dietary regimen that possess a low glycemic index or starch content. A few exemplars include tomatoes, peas, carrots, broccoli, mushrooms, leeks, eggplant, peppers, cauliflower, Brussels sprouts, various greens (such as turnip, mustard, collard, etc.), and bamboo shoots, among others.

Fruits: In a manner similar to vegetables, it is advisable to select fruits that exhibit a low starch or glycemic index. Examples of such fruits include pineapple, mangoes, pears, citrus fruits, dark berries, cherries, apples, oranges, watermelons, and so forth. Purchase fruits that possess a significant amount of hydration.

Animal Protein: Provided that the meat originates from grass-fed animals and is sourced in a sustainable manner, you may incorporate diverse animal-based proteins into your diet, such as whole eggs, poultry, beef, pork, venison, and so forth. Additionally, it is possible to partake in the consumption of seafood items such as shrimp and salmon.

Nutritious Fats: In adhering to a Pegan dietary approach, it is necessary to consume fats derived from minimally processed sources, such as nuts (excluding peanuts), seeds (excluding processed seed oils), unrefined coconut oil, olives, and avocados (ensuring the use of cold-pressed avocado and olive oil). Additionally, incorporating omega-3 fatty acids from low-mercury fish is recommended.

Edible oils and spreads: Due to your dietary restrictions regarding dairy, it is important to note that traditional butter is not suitable for consumption. There exists a multitude of alternatives for butter, ranging from vegan butter to mashed avocado, among other possibilities. Alternatively, various kinds of oils, such as sesame oil and olive oil, can be regarded as examples. Avoid vegetable oils.

Dairy Substitutes: Within the context of a Pegan dietary regimen, one may opt for excellent dairy substitutes such as hemp, almond, soy, cashew, hazelnut, and oat.

Artificial Sweeteners: Incorporating certain organic sources of sugars into your dietary regime is recommended, such as vanilla, dates, honey, coconut sugar, and maple syrup.

Nuts and Seeds: The majority of nuts, such as almonds and walnuts, with the exception of peanuts, are suitable for consumption. When it comes to seeds, one can rely on chia, pumpkin, and flax seeds to add a nutritious boost.

Legumes: While the incorporation of legumes is typically discouraged within the context of the Pegan diet, the consumption of specific gluten-free whole legumes is permitted in constrained amounts. The recommended daily intake should not exceed 75 grams. A few illustrations comprise pinto beans, black beans, chickpeas, and lentils.

Assorted: It is permissible to incorporate an array of diverse ingredients, provided that they possess a low glycemic index value and are of natural origin.

Starches: It is advisable to restrict the consumption of starchy items. Even in the event that you are ingesting starch, it is important to ensure that the origins are nutritionally beneficial.

Bakery goods: When selecting baking supplies, please ensure that the ingredients are free from refined sugar and are suitable for a gluten-free diet. Additionally, you have the option to incorporate black rice, quinoa, oats, black beans, and chickpeas into the mixture.

Supplementary options: When adhering to a Pegan dietary approach, it is possible to incorporate supplementation, such as Vitamin D3 and omega-3 fatty acids. Additionally, you may consider incorporating Vitamin B12 into your supplement regimen.

One-Week Pegan Meal Plan

The Pegan diet places a significant emphasis on the consumption of vegetables and fruits. In addition, this dietary approach incorporates a diverse range of ingredients such as seeds, nuts, seafood, and ethically sourced meats. One may also make limited use of gluten-free grains and select legumes. Herein lies an exemplar menu which you may utilize to prepare meals for the duration of one week:

Monday

Morning meal: Prepare a nutritious vegetable omelet accompanied by a modest green salad, drizzled with olive oil.

Midday Meal: You have the choice of selecting a modest salad comprising avocado, strawberries, and chickpeas.

Tuesday

The day of the week following Tuesday.

Thursday and Friday

Saturday is the forthcoming day of the week.

Dinner can be enjoyed with exceptional choices such as wild salmon patties accompanied by a refreshing lemon vinaigrette, alongside steamed broccoli and roasted carrots, all of which constitute a splendid culinary selection.

Morning Meal: Exercise restraint as you indulge in a delectable sweet potato toast, adorned with a tangy lemon-infused dressing, wholesome pumpkin seeds, and luscious slices of avocado.

Midday Meal: Prepare a traditional Bento box comprising of blackberries, fermented pickles, fresh vegetable batons, turkey slices, and hard-boiled eggs.

Conclude the day with a nutritious evening meal consisting of a vegetable stir-fry prepared with succulent black beans, ripe tomatoes, bell peppers, onions, and delectable cashews.

In the morning, opt for a nutritious and uncomplicated option by preparing a green smoothie containing beneficial ingredients such as hemp seeds, almond butter, kale, and apple.

Lunch: Enjoy a convenient midday meal consisting of the vegetable stir-fry leftovers from Tuesday. Evening meal: Indulge in a sumptuous dining experience featuring delectable vegetable kebabs, grilled shrimp, and a side of black rice pilaf.

Morning Meal: Optimal nourishment for today's breakfast entails indulging in a delectable chia seed and coconut-based pudding, complemented by the presence of succulent blueberries and crunchy walnuts.

Midday Meal: Opting for a mixed green salad dressed with cider vinaigrette, accompanied by grilled chicken, cucumber, and avocado, would be the most favorable selection for today's modest lunch. Dinner: There is the option to choose a delectable roasted beet salad accompanied by sliced almonds, Brussel sprouts, and pumpkin seeds.

Commencing the day with a nourishing breakfast can involve partaking in a combination of braised greens, kimchi, and fried eggs.

Lunch: Opt for a minimalist approach by enjoying a nutritious combination of vegetable stew and lentils, accompanied by a serving of freshly sliced cantaloupe.

Dinner option: Conclude your Friday evening with a nutritious salad consisting of grass-fed beef strips, accompanied by guacamole, jicama, and radishes.

Sunday

Breakfast: Commence your Saturdays by indulging in a nourishing meal of overnight oats, succulent berries, nutritious walnuts, wholesome chia seeds, and rich cashew milk.

Lunch option: Enjoy a serving of yesterday's delectable vegetable stew accompanied by lentils. Evening Meal: Indulge in a splendid Saturday night repast featuring succulent roasted pork loin accompanied by a side of nutritious quinoa, verdant greens, and delectably steamed vegetables.

Morning Meal: Enhance your leisurely Sunday by enjoying a straightforward vegetable omelet accompanied by a refreshing green salad.

Midday Meal: Indulge in the delectable Thai-inspired salad rolls accompanied by segments of fresh orange and a rich cashew cream sauce.

Dinner: Conclude the week by enjoying the pork loin and vegetables from the previous night.

The Advantageous Health Effects Of Adopting The Pegan Diet

A considerable number of individuals who have adhered to the Pegan diet have proclaimed the range of supplementary health benefits in addition to the notion of weight loss or weight management. A few of the additional medical benefits include

included:

Reduced Susceptibility to Cardiovascular Disease

One key advantage of maintaining a well-balanced and intelligent dietary regimen lies in its capacity to promote cardiovascular health. Individuals adhering to a dietary regimen that is abundant in fresh produce derived from whole grains, vegetables, nuts, seeds, and lean proteins appear to possess a significantly reduced likelihood of developing cardiovascular conditions, such as heart failure, stroke, and high blood pressure.

Lowers blood glucose levels.

Multiple studies have demonstrated that adhering to a well-defined, modified, and intelligent dietary regimen can effectively mitigate the risks associated with diabetes and elevated blood glucose levels. Furthermore, in certain instances, this approach has been shown to ameliorate and even reverse type 2 diabetes, obviating the necessity for daily medications.

Diminished Risk of Alzheimer's

Owing to the multitude of cellular benefits associated with consuming a rich variety of fresh food items derived from the source, a consistent adherence to a nutritionally sound regimen has been consistently demonstrated. The risk of an individual developing Alzheimer's disease and other cognitive disorders is diminished.

Weight Reduction

The implementation of limitations on unhealthy food varieties (processed, sugary, or high in unhealthy fats) has demonstrated the positive effects on an individual's body weight, often demonstrating that individuals who adhere to a healthy, balanced, and nourishing diet can achieve long-term weight loss more effectively than their counterparts who do not.

Dietary Options for Consumption on the Pegan Diet

The primary nutritious categorization of the Pegan diet revolves around vegetables and organic produce, comprising 75% of your total dietary consumption. The favorable impact of consuming the soil with low glycemic levels, such as berries and non-starchy vegetables, should be emphasized in order to mitigate the rise in blood sugar levels. Limited quantities of uninteresting vegetables and sweet fruits may be considered for individuals who have successfully achieved stable blood sugar control prior to commencing the diet. Individuals adhering to the Pegan diet are advised to consume meals consisting of whole, minimally processed foods that have remained true to their natural state prior to being prepared in one's kitchen.

"Pegan Diet Buddha Bowl: In Accordance With The Principles Of The Pegan Diet, We Present This Wholesome And Nourishing Buddha Bowl.

INGREDIENTS

- ¼ cup coloured cabbage optional
- 2 onions chopped fine
- 8 cloves garlic minced
- ½ teaspoon Red Chilli powder
- Salt to Taste
- 15-20 cherry tomatoes
- 1 cup carrot sticks
- pumpkin seeds
- 300 grams button mushrooms sauteed
- • 200 grams asparagus sautéed
- 6 boiled eggs
- 1-½ cups quinoa boiled and sautéed
- 1 red capsicum |bell peppers
- ½ zucchini sliced

- 1 head iceberg lettuce

1. Place the mushrooms into a deep pan filled with water in order to thoroughly cleanse away any debris. Bring the water to a boiling point in order to cook the eggs. Thoroughly wash the quinoa and then set it aside. In a sufficiently-sized saucepan, pour in water and bring it to a boiling point. This step is necessary for cooking the quinoa.

2. Let us commence the process of chopping the vegetables. Finely chop two onions and set them aside. Mince the garlic finely and set it aside. Drain the mushrooms and cut them into uniform sizes of either ½ inch or ¼ inch. Chop the broccoli and peel the asparagus.

3. At this point, it is expected that the water intended for cooking the eggs should have reached the boiling point. Transfer the egg into a ladle and carefully submerge it into the boiling

water. I was required to boil a total of six eggs. Allow the eggs to simmer for a duration of 8-10 minutes in order to achieve a hard-boiled consistency. After chilling, remove the peel and set it aside.

4. Introduce the quinoa into the boiling water, along with a pinch of salt for flavor, and thoroughly combine the ingredients. Maintain a low flame and allow the quinoa to simmer. The grains are considered cooked once the Germ Check is visibly detectable. For more comprehensive information on the process of boiling quinoa, please refer to the link provided within the notes section.

5. Incorporate salt, garlic, and approximately 3 tablespoons of onions into the mushrooms, along with chili powder. Proceed by setting this mixture aside.

6. In the interim, proceed to strain the eggs whilst incorporating the broccoli into the same pan. Add a small amount

of water and salt, subsequently steaming the broccoli.

7. Incorporate the garlic and 1 teaspoon of olive oil into a saucepan, and cook until the pungent aroma dissipates. Integrate the asparagus into the mixture and sauté until fully cooked. Set aside.

8. Incorporate the mushrooms into the same pan and cook until they are fully sautéed. Set aside

9. Incorporate 1 tablespoon of oil and proceed to sauté the remaining garlic and onions. Incorporate the chilled quinoa and sauté. Set aside.

Tagliatelle With Salmon

ingredients

50ml white wine
dill to taste
freshly ground black pepper to taste
Salt to taste.
320 g egg tagliatelle pasta
160 g smoked salmon
2 tablespoons of extra virgin olive oil
1 sprig of parsley
1 shallot

Preparation

Place a sizable cooking vessel onto the stovetop, ensuring that it is filled with an ample amount of water, and proceed to heat it until it reaches its boiling point. In the interim, slice the salmon into strips of appropriate size, ensuring they are not excessively small so as to maintain their structural integrity while being cooked. Thoroughly mince the shallot and parsley. Position a substantial skillet onto the heat source, incorporate the extra virgin olive oil, and allow it to reach an elevated temperature for a brief duration. Subsequently, introduce the finely chopped shallot and allow it to desiccate without undergoing any change in coloration, employing a medium intensity flame. Incorporate the salmon into the mixture, and if the fragrance is to your liking, consider adding a small amount of dill. Sear the ingredients for a brief duration and combine to preference with a white wine (or, if preferred, substitute with brandy, white rum, vodka, or even champagne), allowing for complete evaporation. In order to eliminate the need for cream, it is necessary to properly prepare the pasta by thoroughly stirring it as it cooks, allowing it to release its starch content.

Upon cooking the tagliatelle in water seasoned with salt, remove it from heat while it is still firm to the bite, and ensure the preservation of the cooking water at a warm temperature, aside from the pasta. Transfer the pasta into the pan containing the shallot and salmon mixture, stir and proceed with the cooking process by gradually incorporating the cooking water, mimicking the technique employed in the preparation of risotto. This method will yield a lusciously smooth and delectable dish. Furthermore, during this stage, it is important to include a dash of freshly ground black pepper and finely cut parsley. Combine using wooden utensils and, after thorough stirring, promptly serve the salmon tagliatelle while it is still hot.

1onion Millet

Ingredients:

.

- ½ cup millet
- ½ teaspoon ground black pepper
- 1 cup vegetable broth
- ½ tablespoon vegetable oil
- 1 red onion, chopped

Directions:

1. Warm the oil in the Instant Pot using the Sauté function. Incorporate the

onion and continue cooking until it reaches a tender consistency. Incorporate millet into the mixture and continue cooking until it is fully coated with oil. When the onion has reached a tender consistency and the millet has lightly browned, proceed to season with pepper and carefully pour in the vegetable stock. Securely seal the Instant Pot by adjusting the tension valve to the Sealing position. Set the cooking mode to Manual for a duration of 10 minutes, then proceed with a regular 10-minute natural pressure release.

2. Open Instant Pot.

3. Enjoy.

Zucchini Ribbons With Sautéed Shrimp In A Garlic-Infused Butter Sauce

Ingredients

- 1 tbsp. minced garlic
- 2 medium spiralized zucchinis
- 2 tbsps. freshly squeezed lemon juice
- Chopped parsley

- 2 tbsps. olive oil
- 1lb. peeled and deveined jumbo shrimp
- ¼ tsp. crushed red-pepper flakes
- ¼ c. white wine

Instructions

Arrange a frying pan and heat it with oil. Incorporate finely minced garlic and a dash of red chili flakes.

Allow them to cook for a minute, all the while stirring incessantly.

Incorporate the shrimp into the pan and cook them while intermittently stirring for approximately 3 minutes or until fully cooked.

Season the shrimp with seasonings and transfer them to a bowl using a slotted spoon, ensuring any excess liquid remains in the pan.

Set the heat to a moderate level and incorporate lemon juice and white wine into the pan. Remove any lightly browned residue from the pan and proceed to cook the wine and lemon juice for a duration of approximately two minutes.

Incorporate zucchini noodles into the mixture; allow them to cook for approximately 2 minutes. Return the shrimp to the pan and gently mix until thoroughly combined.

Include spices and herbs, followed by the addition of freshly chopped parsley for garnish.

Serve immediately and enjoy.

Morning Porridge Filled With Nuts

Ingredients

- 2 tablespoons stevia
- 4 teaspoons coconut oil, melted
- 2 cups of water
- 1 cup cashew nuts, raw and unsalted
- 1 cup pecan, halved

Directions

Process the nuts in a food processor until they attain a creamy consistency.

Combine water, oil, and stevia with the nuts paste, then transfer the mixture to a saucepan.

Heat the mixture on high for 5 minutes, stirring continuously.

Lower heat to low and simmer for 10 minutes

Please kindly indulge in this dish while it is still warm.

Collard Green Omelet

Ingredients:

- 4 large eggs
- ½-inch piece American pancetta or 4 oz bacon, diced
- ¼ cup vegetable stock, or chicken stock, water
- Chopped fresh parsley
- A pinch of salt
- A pinch of black pepper, ground
- A few drops of chipotle hot sauce, or favored hot sauce
- Dash of chardonnay vinegar
- 3 tbsp unsalted butter, separated into individual tablespoons
- 1 lb baby hearty greens (beet greens, collard greens, dandelion greens, or mustard greens), remove stems if needed

Directions:

In a single pan, heat and melt one tablespoon of butter over a medium flame.

• Place the pancetta or bacon into the pan and cook for approximately 10 minutes, or until it reaches a crispy consistency.

• Incorporate the preferred selection of greens into the mixture, along with stock or water, vinegar, and hot sauce.

• Simmer the greens in this concoction for approximately five minutes or until they have reached a state of gentle wilting.

• Incorporate additional stock or water if the greens become too dry prior to achieving tenderness.

• Add a dash of salt and pepper to enhance the flavors.

In a separate pan, place 2 tablespoons of butter and heat until it reaches a simmering point.

Whisk the eggs vigorously until they achieve a fluffy consistency, followed by adding a dash of salt and pepper.

● Incorporate the egg mixture into the pan and allow it to cook for approximately one minute until the lower layer is beginning to solidify.

● Gently lift the rim of the well-cooked egg and create an opening for the uncooked portion to seamlessly distribute beneath.

● Proceed to repeat the process with each edge of the cooked egg until all residual liquid egg has been completely cooked.

● Place the cooked greens at the center of the omelet and proceed to roll it into a cylindrical shape.

- Transfer the omelet onto a plate and generously sprinkle it with salt and pepper, garnished with a sprinkle of parsley.

Paleo-Inspired Skillet Sausage Hash Accompanied By Eggs

- 1/2 tsp paprika, garlic powder, and a dash of cumin
- 4 eggs
- A handful of chopped green onion or scallions

- **Kosher salt, pepper**

- 3 tbsp refined coconut oil
- 3 sweet potatoes, chopped in 1/2 chunks
- 1 medium white onion, chopped
- 1 garlic clove, minced
- 1 medium bell pepper, chopped
- 1/2 pound ground sausage or ground turkey

Set the oven temperature to 400 degrees Fahrenheit prior to usage. We will utilize it for the purpose of cooking the eggs at a later time.

Preheat your preferred cast-iron skillet or oven-safe pan using one tablespoon of coconut oil. Break up the sausage into smaller pieces and mix it into the pan. Cook over medium-high heat. Incorporate the garlic powder, paprika, and a small amount of cumin.

After the sausage has reached a state of 75% cooked, incorporate the onions, bell peppers, and garlic.

Place the sweet potatoes in a microwave-safe bowl and heat them on high for a duration of 5 minutes, as this will expedite the process of softening them. Agitate the contents of the bowl at the midpoint.

Transfer the heated sweet potatoes into a distinct small skillet, along with the remaining coconut oil. Incorporate paprika and garlic powder. Cook until a deep, rich golden hue is achieved, typically requiring approximately 5 minutes.

Integrate the sausage, vegetables, and sweet potato into the cast iron skillet. Using the rear side of a spoon, fashion four indentations in the pan to accommodate the eggs, and subsequently, shatter each egg directly into the pan.

Place the skillet in the oven for approximately 10 minutes or until the eggs are cooked to your desired level of doneness. Savour the dish accompanied by finely minced green onion and a sprinkling of red pepper flakes.

Nutty Toasted 'Cereal'

- 1/3 cup maple syrup
- 1/3 cup coconut oil
- 1 tsp cinnamon
- 2 tsp vanilla
- 1 cup dried cranberries
- 1 cup chopped dried apricots

- **1 cup golden raisins**

- 1 1/2 cups pumpkin seeds
- 1 cup sunflower seeds
- 1 1/2 cups sliced almonds
- 1 1/2 cups chopped pecans
- 1 1/2 unsweetened shredded coconut

Set the oven to a temperature of 375 degrees Fahrenheit in advance. Prepare a baking sheet by covering it with parchment paper, and then set it aside.

Incorporate pumpkin seeds, sunflower seeds, almonds, pecans, and coconut in a substantial-sized bowl.

Using a small saucepan, gently heat the maple syrup and coconut oil until the oil has completely melted. Take away from the source of heat and incorporate cinnamon and vanilla by stirring. Transfer the mixture into the bowl containing the nuts, and proceed to blend it meticulously, ensuring that all components are uniformly coated.

Evenly distribute the mixture onto the baking sheet using a rubber spatula. Spread evenly.

Place in the oven and bake for a duration of 20 to 30 minutes, ensuring to stir delicately every ten minutes. Nuts ought to be gently toasted, exhibiting a light brown hue and exuding a pleasing aroma.

Take out from the oven and incorporate cranberries, apricots, and raisins by stirring. Allow all contents to cool naturally, intermittently stirring, for approximately 20 minutes.

Place in a hermetically sealed receptacle at ambient temperature for a maximum duration of three weeks.

Braised Artichokes Accompanied By Peas And Potatoes

INGREDIENTS

- 150 ml broth or water
- aromatic herbs to taste
- 10 walnuts
- 2 tablespoons flaxseed
- Himalayan pink salt and pepper
- 300 g artichoke hearts
- 2 nuts of avocado butter or coconut oil
- 1 leek
- 1 clove of garlic
- 270 g potatoes (new potatoes are better if you can)
- 250 g peas

PROCEDURE

1. Commence the process by thoroughly cleansing the leek, subsequently slicing it into circular pieces. Proceed by removing the shells from the walnuts, followed by finely chopping them. Concurrently, cleanse and finely chop the herbs as well. Prepare the potatoes by removing the outer skin and cutting them into small cube-shaped pieces. In a cooking pan, proceed to heat the butter and subsequently incorporate the garlic and leek. Allow them to gently soften, and then introduce the prepared potato cubes into the pan.

2. Incorporate a small amount of broth and proceed to simmer with the lid secured for approximately 6 minutes. Subsequently, incorporate the sliced artichoke hearts into wedges, peas, and the remaining portion of broth. Place a lid over the pot and allow the mixture to cook over a moderate heat until the

potatoes and artichokes have achieved a tender consistency (if needed, you may add water and prolong the cooking duration).

3. Immediately prior to discontinuing the application of heat, lightly sprinkle salt and pepper, incorporate the herbs, finely diced walnuts, and flaxseed. Thoroughly mix to season and subsequently influence! Furthermore, this dish can be enjoyed at a low temperature.

Maple-Pegan Macaroons

Ingredients

- 2 cups (170 g) finely shredded unsweetened coconut
- ½ cup (55 g) finely chopped pecans, plus more for garnish (optional)
- 3 ounces (85 g) unsweetened chocolate
- ⅓ cup (107 g) maple syrup
- 1 teaspoon grass-fed gelatin
- ½ teaspoon almond exact
- ½ teaspoon vanilla extract

Directions

Kindly ensure that the oven is set to a preheating temperature of 350°F (180°C, or gas mark 4). Prepare a baking sheet by placing a layer of parchment paper or a silicone baking mat onto it.

In a bowl of moderate size, vigorously stir together the egg whites and maple syrup until achieving a highly foamy consistency. There is no requirement to vigorously whisk the mixture until peaks are formed, as is typically done when making meringue. However, it is important for the mixture to achieve a discernibly lighter consistency.

Incorporate the gelatin, almond extract, and vanilla into the mixture, whisking thoroughly.

Incorporate the coconut and pecans into the mixture, ensuring they are thoroughly coated with the egg white mixture.

Employ a spherical tablespoon or cookie scoop to draw out and compress the coconut batter, applying pressure to achieve a cohesive consistency, prior to positioning it atop the prearranged baking sheet. Produce an additional batch to yield a total of 20 cookies.

Place the cookies in the oven and allow them to bake for a duration of 16 to 18 minutes, or until a light golden brown hue has been achieved on the surface. Let cool fully.

Dissolve the unsweetened chocolate using a double boiler. Immerse the bottom of every cookie into the liquefied chocolate for an even coating, gently transferring them onto a sheet of wax paper to solidify. Utilize a utensil such as a fork to slowly distribute any excess

chocolate drizzled atop the cookies. Add a sprinkling of additional chopped pecans onto the cookies, if desired.

Coconut Banana Cream Pie

INGREDIENTS

- 3tablespoons unsalted butter
- 2 teaspoons vanilla
- 3 teaspoons coconut extract divided
- 3 cups shredded sweetened coconut divided
- 2 medium bananas sliced
- 1 1/2 cups whipping cream, chilled
- 3 tablespoons powdered sugar
- 1all-butter pie crust from a pack of two or a homemade crust
- 3/4 cup sugar
- 1/4 cup cornstarch
- 1/2 teaspoon salt
- 3cups whole milk
- 2eggs lightly beaten

For the preparation of single-crust pudding pie, kindly adhere to the instructions provided by the manufacturer or follow the guidelines outlined in the recipe. Allow to cool.

Incorporate the sugar, salt, cornstarch, and milk in a medium saucepan. Gently heat the mixture, continuously whisking or stirring, over medium-high heat until it reaches a thick and bubbling consistency (approximately 7-8 minutes). Reduce the heat to low and continue cooking for an additional 2 minutes.

A minuscule amount of the warmed milk mixture should be incorporated into the lightly whisked eggs. To prevent the eggs from becoming scrambled, it is essential to continuously whisk throughout the process. Replenish the pan with the mixture of milk and beaten eggs. Proceed to heat until boiling, then continue cooking for an additional 2 minutes, while frequently stirring. When the item is reintroduced into the pan, it will rapidly reach boiling point.

Incorporating the butter, vanilla extract, and 2 teaspoons of coconut extract into the pudding once it has been removed from the heat. Through the process of carefully sieving the pudding into a suitable receptacle, one can ensure the absence of any residual traces of egg.

Add 2 cups of shredded coconut to the mixture, and repeat this step for a total of 2 cups.

Proceed by refrigerating the mixture for a minimum of 30 minutes, up to a maximum of 24 hours, before serving.

Commence the process of pie assembly by carefully spreading a delicate layer of cushioning on the base of the crust. Finish by layering the remaining pudding and a singular stratum of diced bananas on top. Place the pie in the refrigerator and allow it to chill for a minimum of two hours, ideally overnight.

Using a saucepan with a sturdy base, placed over gentle heat, proceed to brown the remaining quarter cup of coconut. You must stir the mixture constantly until the coconut achieves a golden color. Expeditiously removing the pan from the heat is a prudent course of action. During the process of cooking, it is crucial to closely monitor the coconut as it has a tendency to rapidly toast and char.

Prepare the whipped cream immediately prior to serving. In order to utilize an electric mixer, vigorously whip the heavy whipping cream until it reaches a consistency of firm peaks. Proceed with adding 1 teaspoon of coconut essence and powdered sugar in a gradual manner. Beat the cream with an electrical mixer until it reaches the consistency of stiff peaks. Topped with toasted coconut and whipped cream, the pie is delicious. Please ensure that the service is provided within the upcoming 48 hours.

www.ingramcontent.com/pod-product-compliance
Lightning Source LLC
Chambersburg PA
CBHW071213020426
42333CB00015B/1399